How To Use Beeswax and Honey to Cure Skin Problems

By
Gene Ashburner

Second Edition 2018

ISBN-13:978-1503084926
ISBN-10:1503084922

Content

Second Edition 2018

ISBN-13:978-1503084926
ISBN-10:1503084922

Content

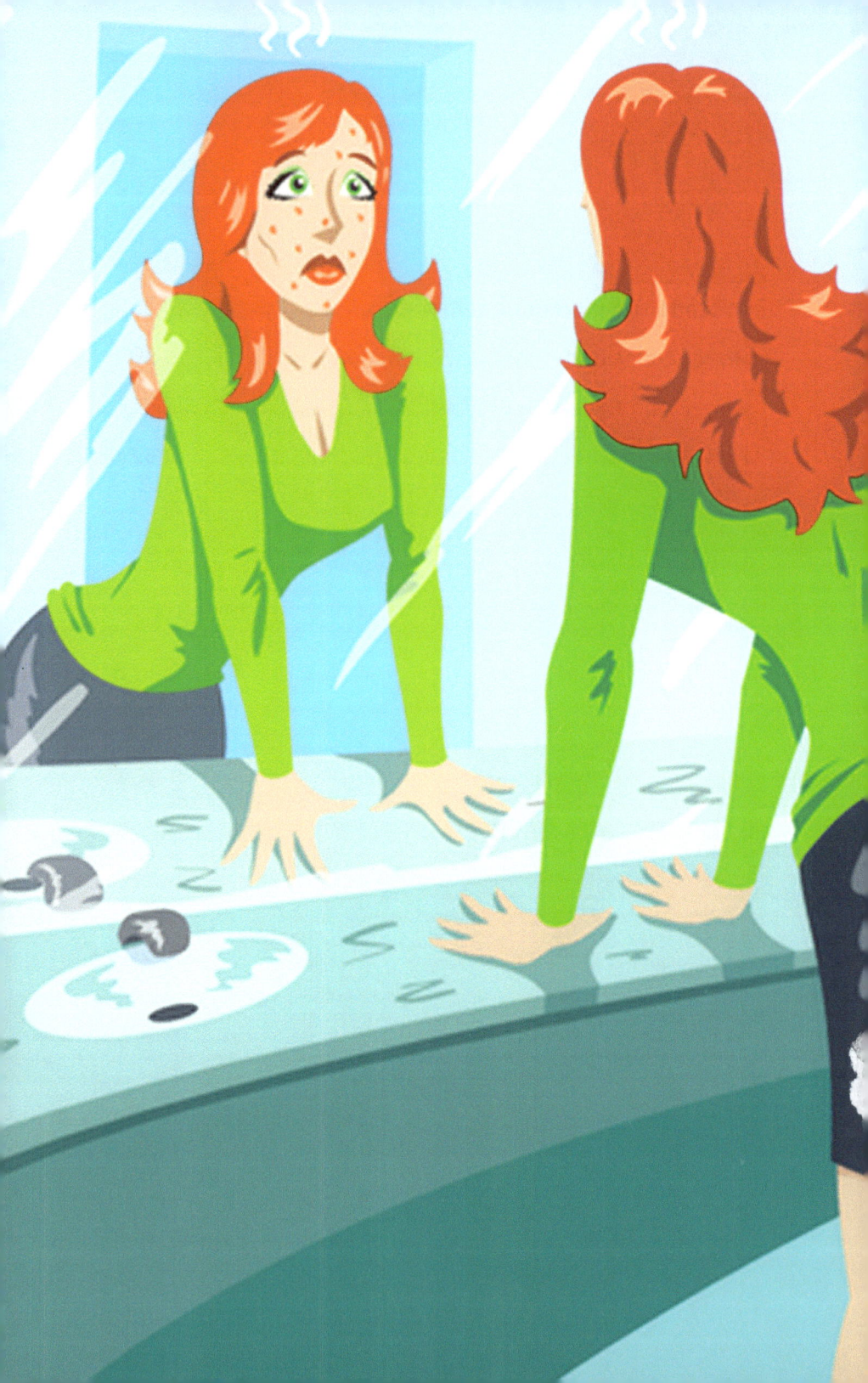

How To Use Beeswax And Honey To Cure Skin Problems

I have always had a problem skin!! Expensive skin products just didn't work for my skin. In fact nothing worked....

I had assumed if I bought expensive products I would solve the problem but it didn't work out like that !!!

I was desperate so I started looking around for natural products and remedies. I had got to the stage where my skin was scarred from all the years of skin problems so I was looking for something that would heal my skin and also prevent further skin problems and breakouts.

In this book I will show you what I discovered and how well it worked!!

This is What My Skin Looked Like Before I Started Looking For A Natural Product Solution

1) Brown patches and blemishes

2) Blackheads and whiteheads

3) Uneven skin tone

4) Pimples

5) Scars

6) Dry scaly skin in parts and oily skin in other parts

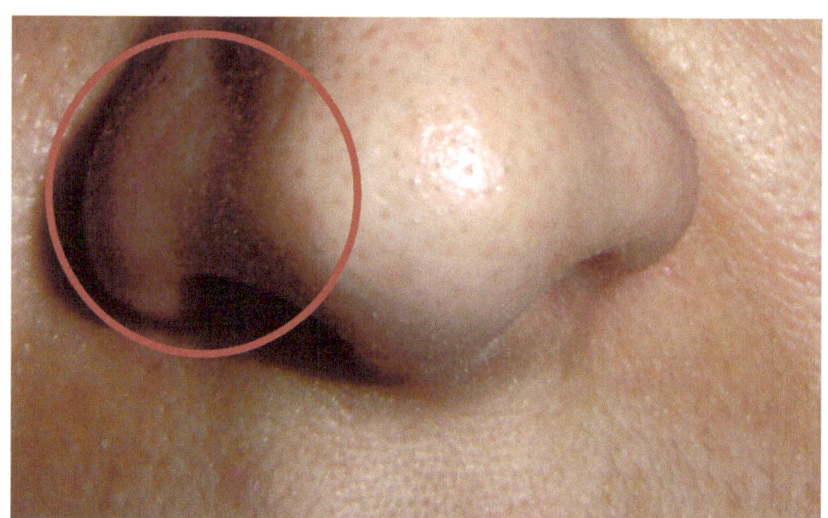

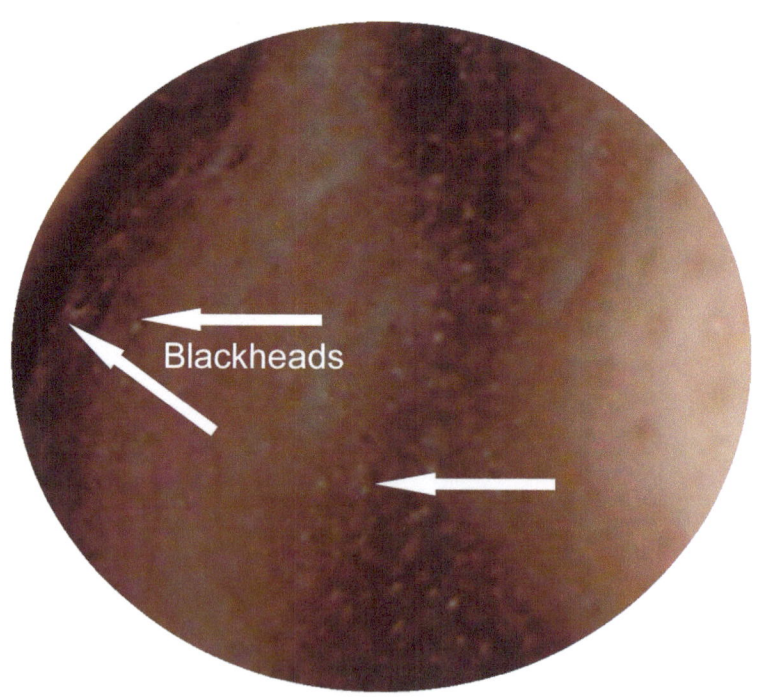

Blackheads

This Is What My Skin Looks Like Now – 6 Months Later

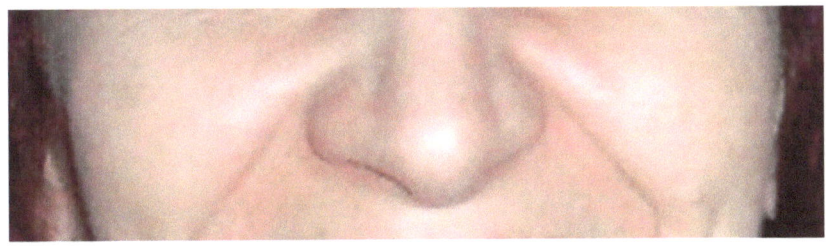

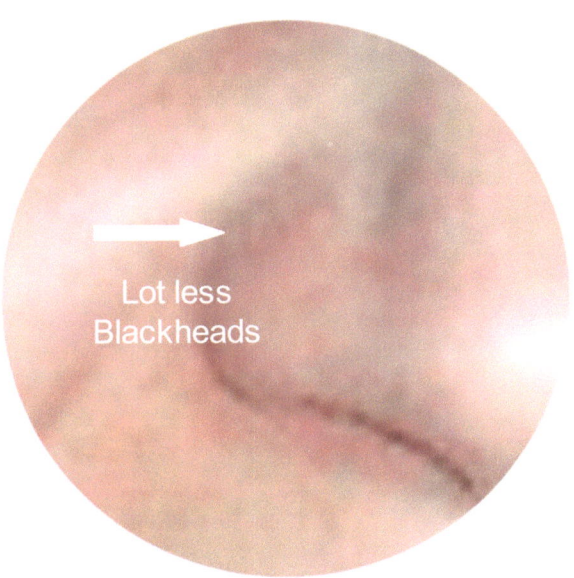

So What Was My Solution?

It was such a simple solution!!!

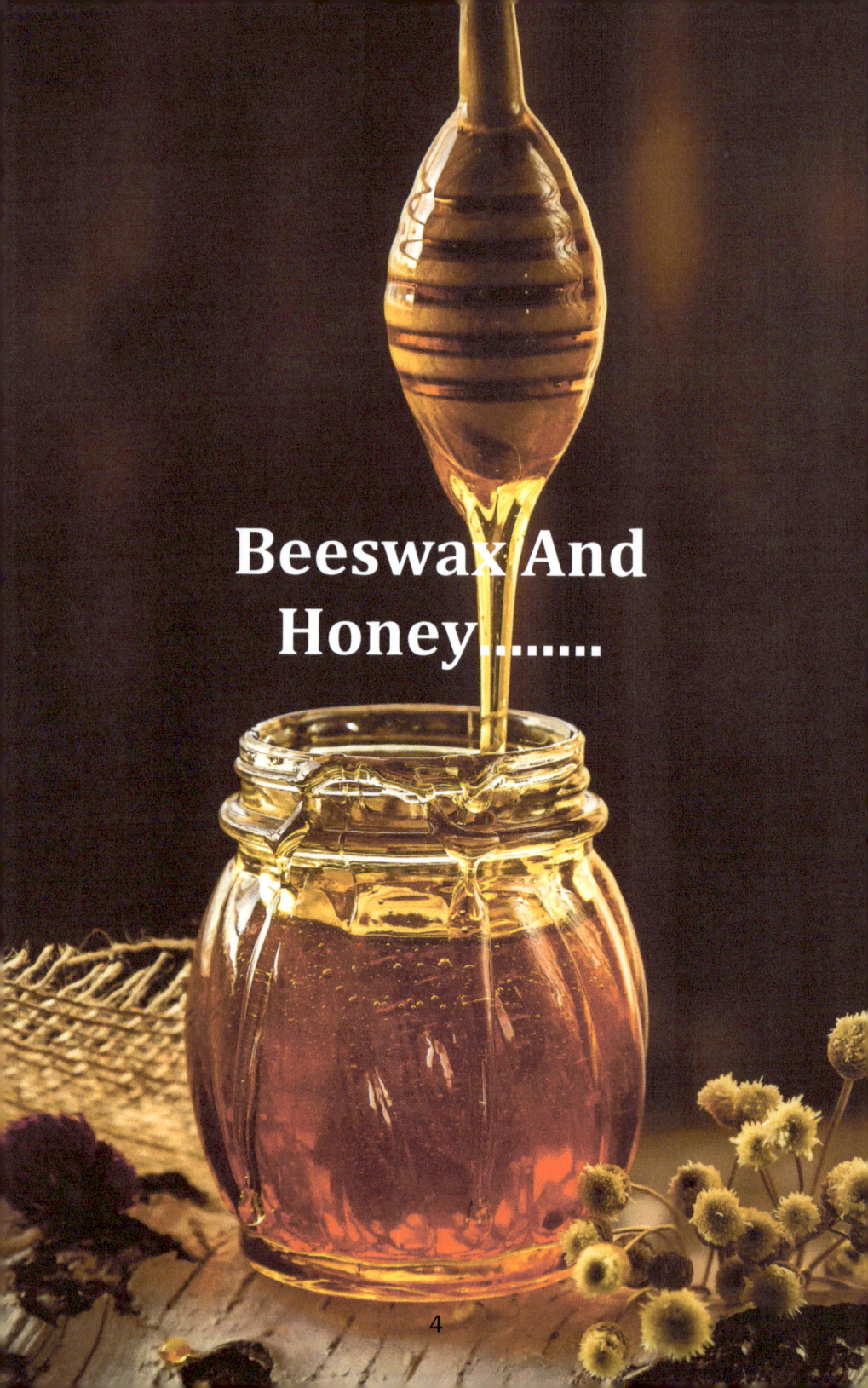

Beeswax And
Honey........

This Is What My Skin Looks Like Now – 6 Months Later

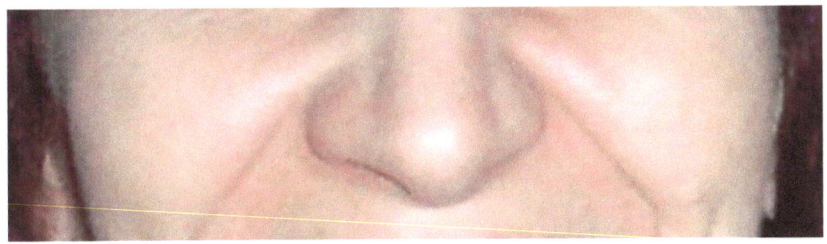

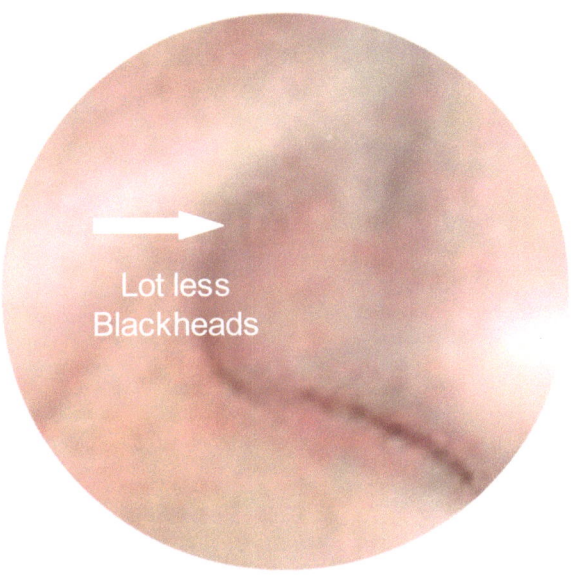

So What Was My Solution?

It was such a simple solution!!!

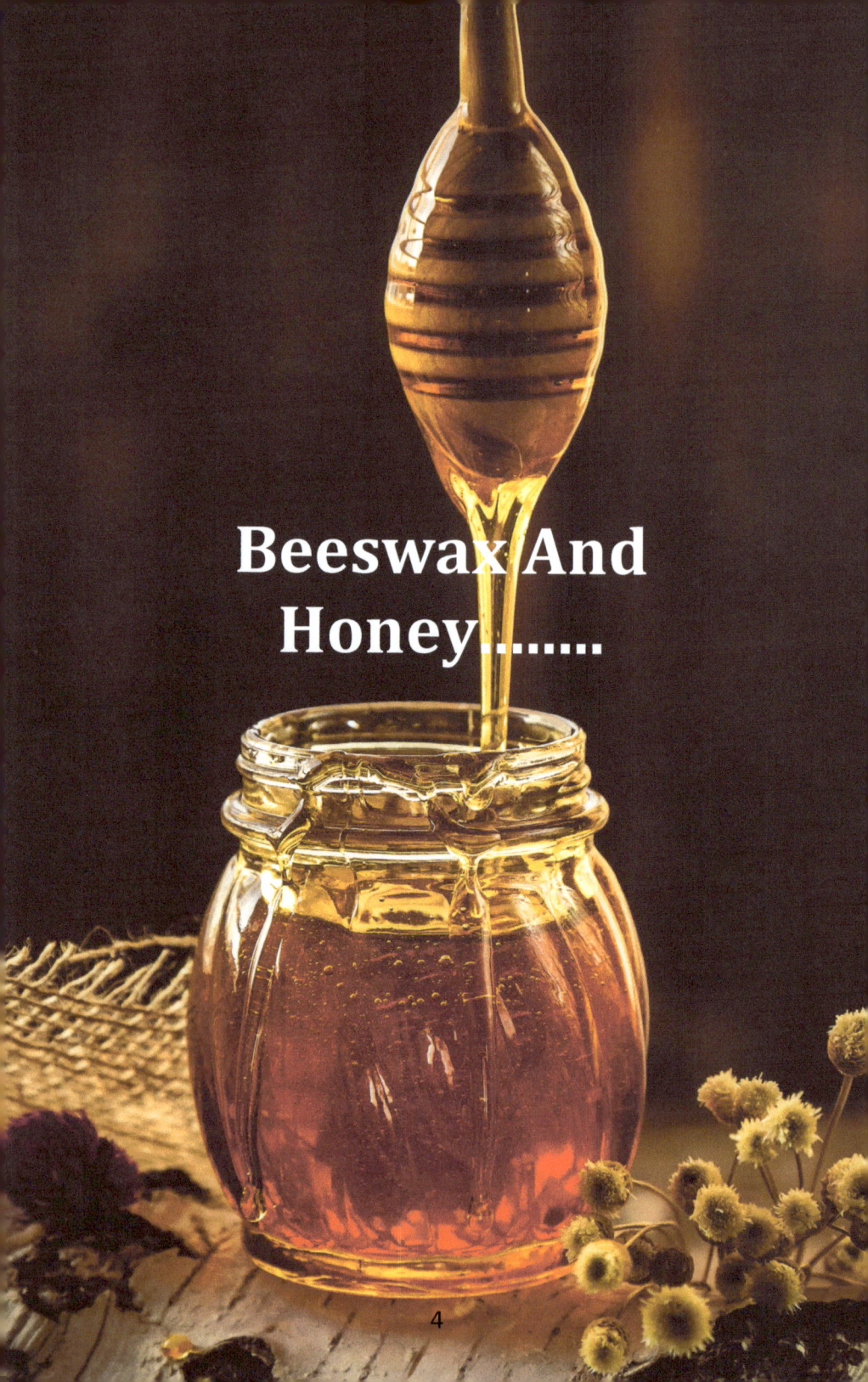

Beeswax And Honey.......

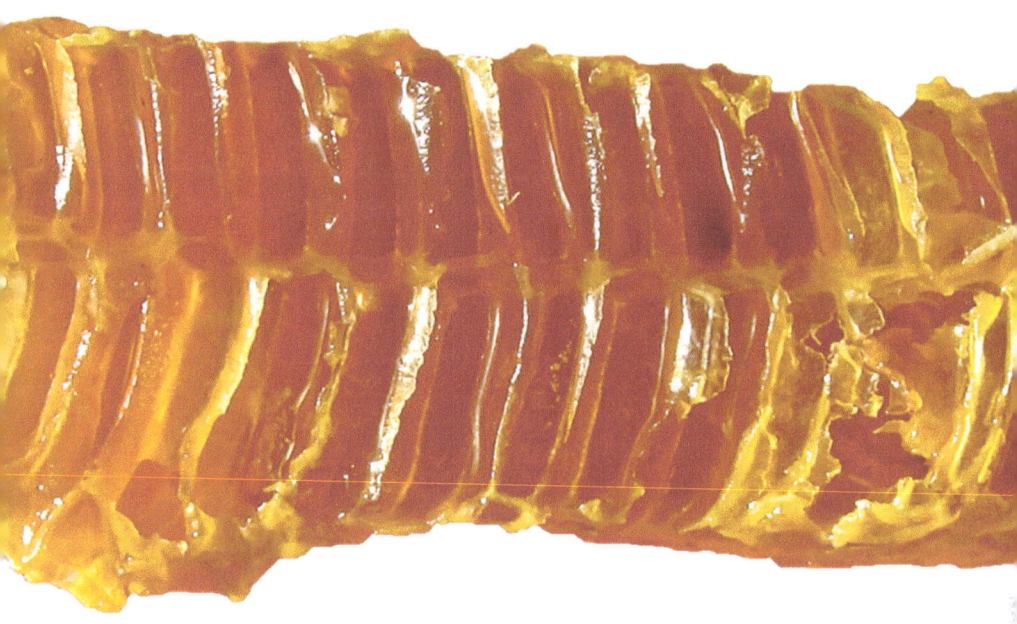

Why beeswax?

I discovered that beeswax has the following qualities and benefits...

Beeswax is a natural product and is totally non toxic and known for its healing properties.

> beeswax is anti-inflammatory - helps encourage the healing of wounds
>
> beeswax is antibacterial
>
> beeswax is anti-allergenic
>
> beeswax is a germicidal antioxidant

Beeswax contains vitamin A which is necessary for normal cell development.

Beeswax feels incredibly good on your skin because it softens and rehydrates the skin while aiding cellular reconstruction.

Because of comedogenicity beeswax does not clog pores while it seals in the moisturizing oils and butters.

Beeswax creates a long-lasting protective coating against the elements.

Beeswax works very well in sunscreens because of its water repellent properties.

Beeswax has been found to be superior to barrier creams such as mineral oil based creams.

Beeswax is Humectant – this means it attracts water molecules which when put onto your skin will keep your skin hydrated over time.

Beeswax alleviates itching – prefect for dry skin itching, dermatitis, eczema or any type of itching related to a skin condition.

Post-burn Itch – people with serious burns experience relief when using beeswax based lotions.

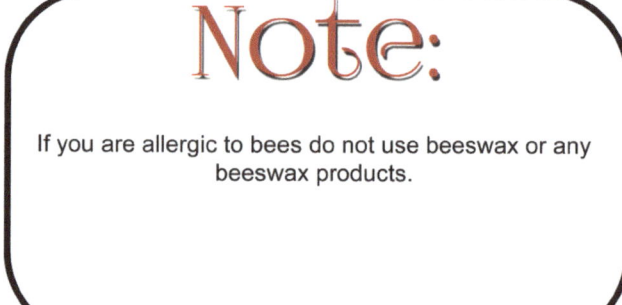

Note:

If you are allergic to bees do not use beeswax or any beeswax products.

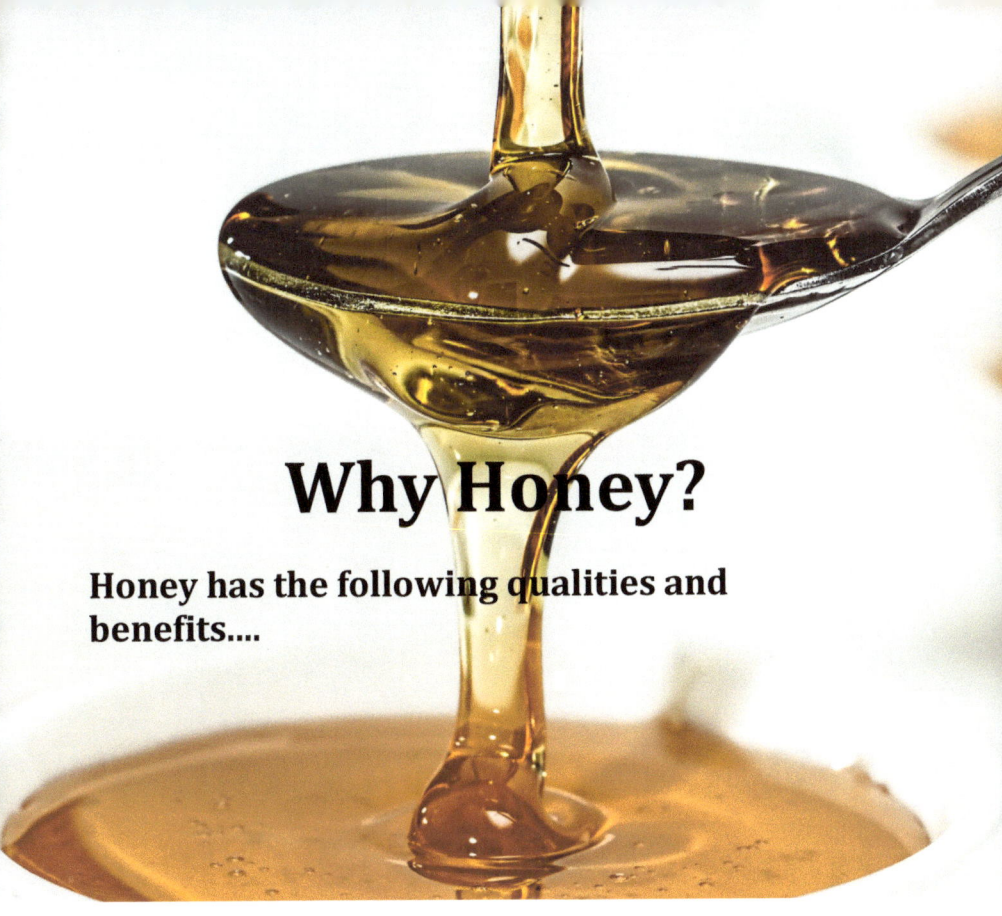

Why Honey?

Honey has the following qualities and benefits....

Reduces acne

Reduces the size of enlarged pores

Can be used for skin problems such as Rosacea and Eczema

Hyper pigmentation

Improves the quality of mature and lifeless skin

Honey contains anti-microbial properties and natural antioxidants

Honey prevents the breakout of blackheads

Note:

If you are allergic to bees do not use beeswax or any beeswax products.

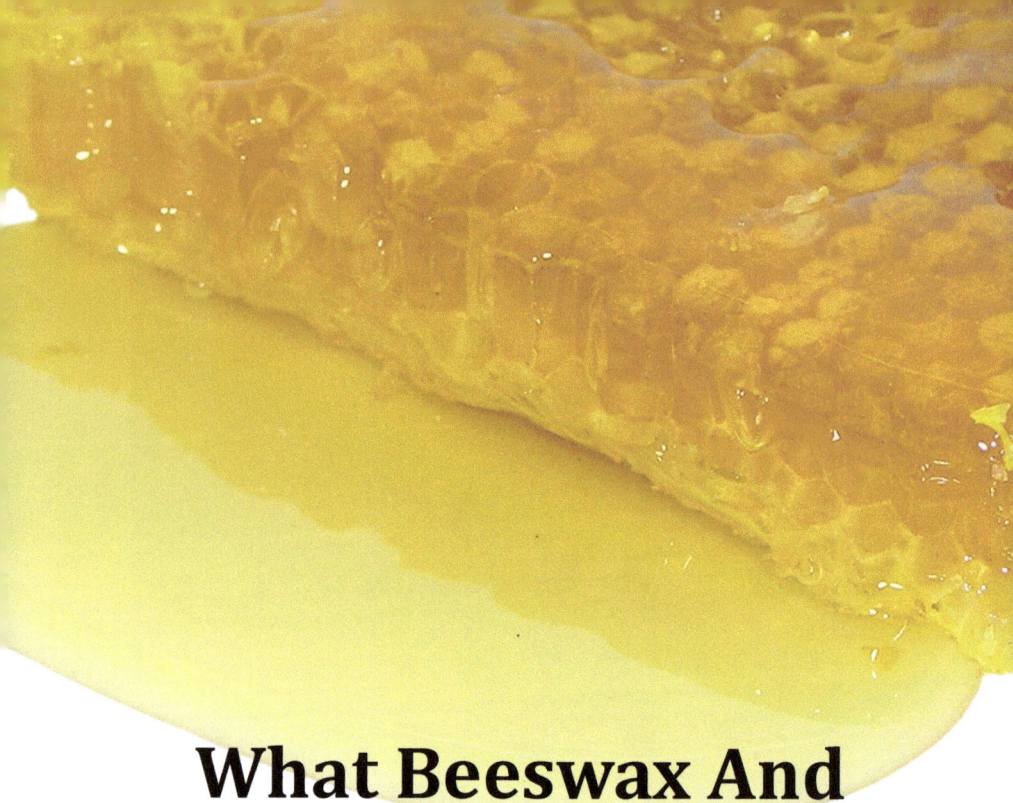

What Beeswax And Honey Did For My Skin

Removed dark spots and blemishes from my skin

Removed deep lines from my forehead

Tightened the enlarged pores

Brought out whiteheads that were not visible but made unsightly bumps under my skin and never seemed to heal

Moisturised my skin

Improved the texture of my skin

The appearance of pimples and blackheads lessened as the time went by

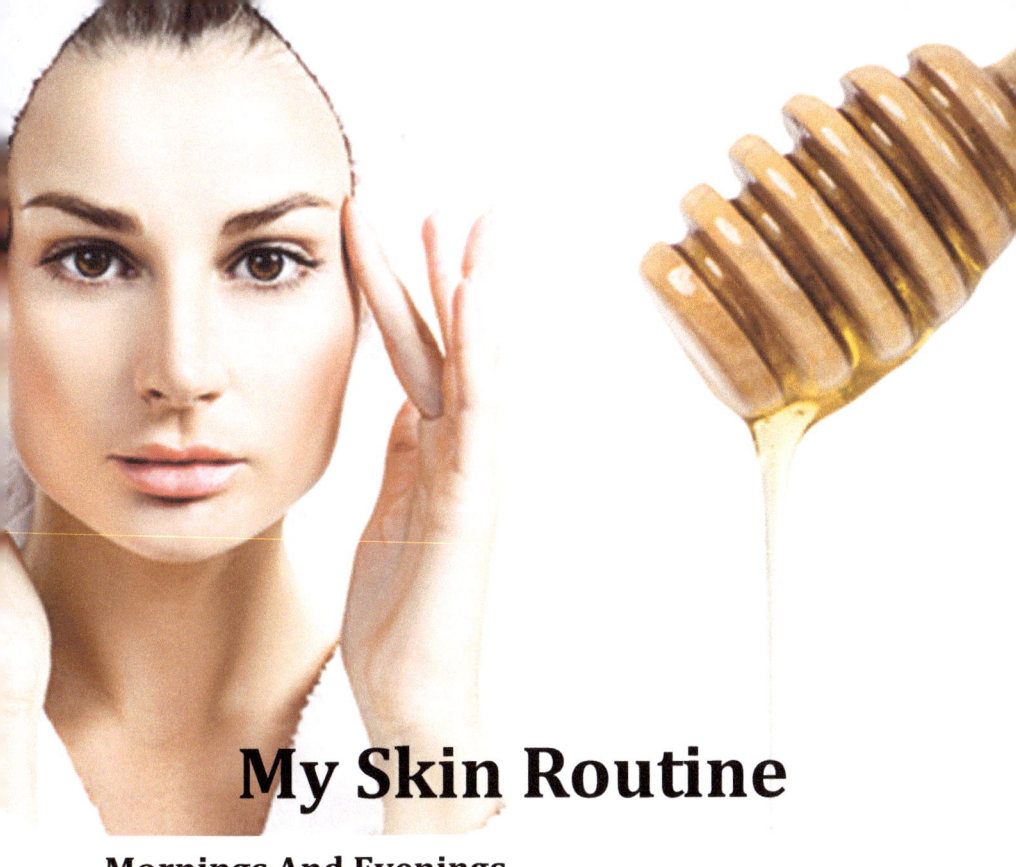

My Skin Routine

Mornings And Evenings

I wash my face with Honey and Glycerin Soap (Recipe in the back of the book).

I then apply Beeswax Moisturizer onto my newly cleaned skin (Recipe in the back of the book).

Weekly

I apply the Honey Apple Face Mask once per week (Recipe in the back of the book).

Miscellaneous

1) The Honey Pimple Remedy is great for the occasional pimple outbreak (Recipe in the back of the book).

2) I have included recipes for hand and body lotions, body butter and body scrubs.

Beeswax Body Butter

Beeswax Lotion Bars

Beeswax Hand Lotion

Honey Almond Sugar Scrub

Honey Pistachio Sugar Scrub

3) I have also included recipes for hair products

Avocado Honey Hair Conditioner

Honey Hair Conditioner

Honey And Banana Hair Mask

Honey Hair Mask

Honey Shampoo

4) There are also lip products to keep your lips soft and supple.

Beeswax Lip Balm

Beeswax Lip Gloss

Making Your Own Beeswax And Honey Products

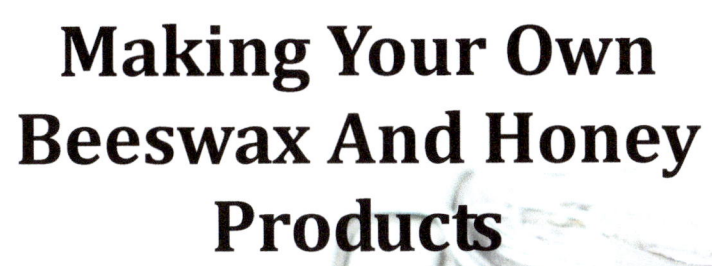

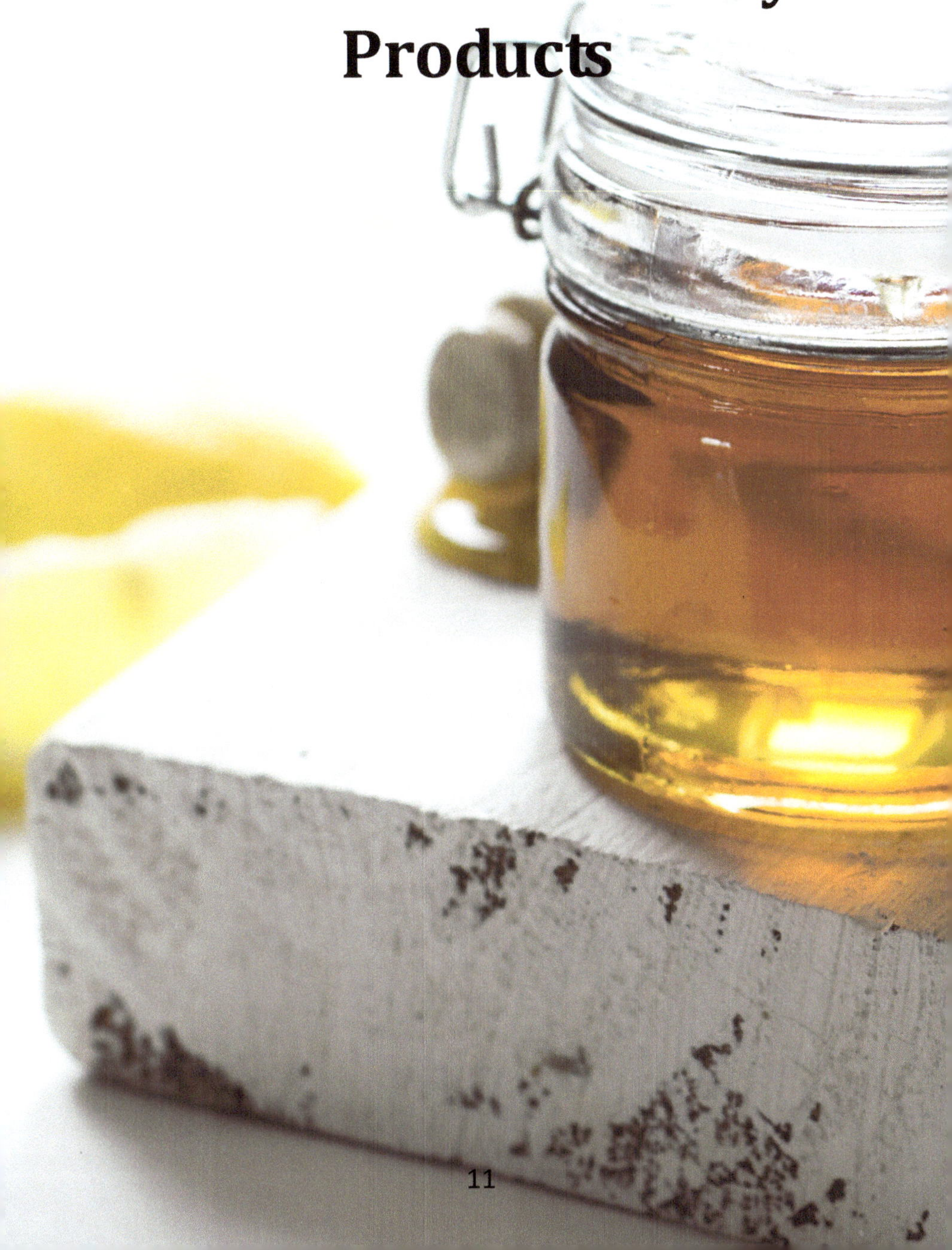

Types Of Beeswax – What Is The Difference?

Beeswax starts off being white and then turns yellow with age. This is due to propolis and pollen oil incorporation.

Blended Beeswax

Other waxes are mixed with the beeswax (for example paraffin). You would use this if you were making beeswax candles and wanted a longer burning candle.

Bleached Beeswax

This is known as ivory beeswax and can be bleached by the sun or chemical bleaching.

This type of beeswax is odorless and used in candles or commercial cosmetics.

Raw Bees wax

Raw beeswax contains particles and residue due to the absence of any refining process.

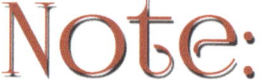

Note:

You do not want to use chemical processed beeswax when making your natural beeswax products.

How To Melt Beeswax

Equipment Requited

A double boiler such as the one below. This type of double boiler can be placed into a standard sized saucepan. You can also buy double boilers that have their own saucepan included.

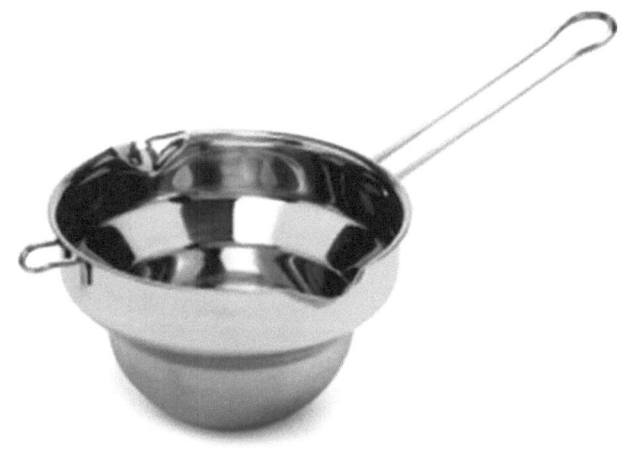

Method

Place water into the bottom part of the double boiler.

Bring the water to boiling point.

Turn the temperature down so that the water remains at a simmer.

Place the beeswax into the top part of the double boiler.

Place the top part of the boiler containing the beeswax onto of the simmering water.

Allow the beeswax to melt and reach the required temperature (62 to 64 °C).

Note:

Never melt the beeswax directly on the stove (it could scorch the beeswax or cause a fire).

The melting point range of beeswax is 62 to 64 °C

The flash point of beeswax is 204.4 °C

Beeswax will discolor if heated above 85 °C

Beeswax Body Product Recipes

You should use natural beeswax whenever possible, it should not be chemically bleached, deodorized or chemically treated in any way.

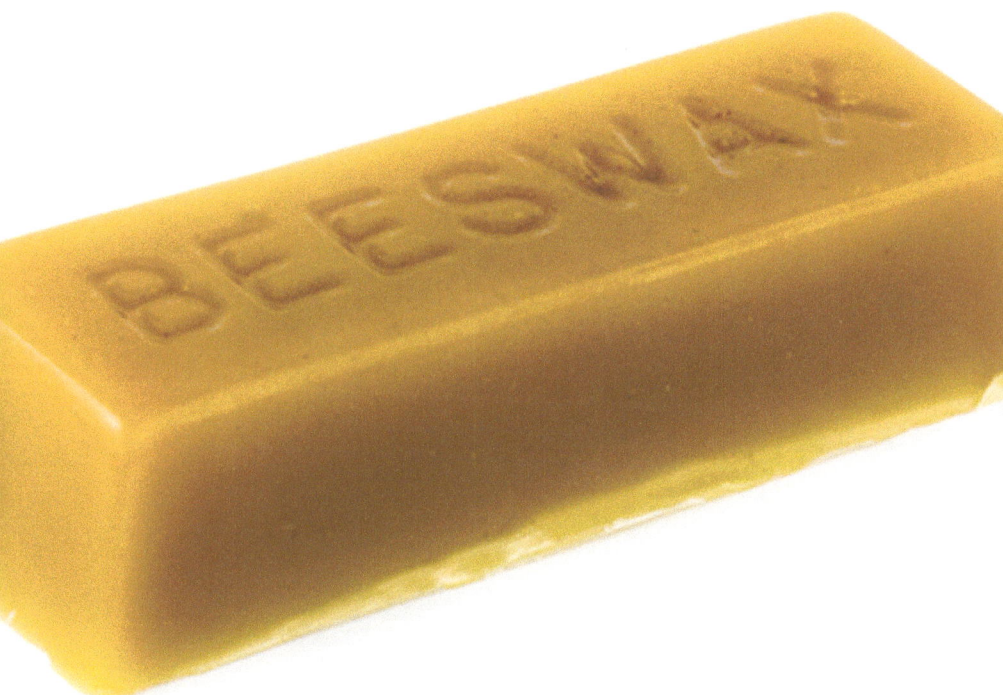

Beeswax Moisturizer

Ingredients

187 ml beeswax

187 ml olive oil

375 ml coconut oil

20 ml honey

Method

Combine the beeswax, olive oil and coconut oil together in the top of a double boiler over boiling water.

Mix well.

Once the oils have melted remove from the heat.

Add the honey.

Mix well.

Pour the hot mixture into a sterilized jar.

Leave the moisturizer to set.

Beeswax Body Butter

Ingredients

250 ml beeswax

250 ml petroleum jelly

250 ml almond oil

250 ml honey

50 ml bee pollen

250 ml glycerin

50 ml liquid lecithin

Method

Melt the beeswax and petroleum jelly together in the top of a double boiler over boiling water.

Mix well.

Once the mixture has melted add the almond oil, honey, bee pollen, glycerine and liquid lecithin.

Mix well and heat for 5 minutes.

Mix until smooth.

Remove the mixture from the heat.

Scoop the body butter into a sterilized container and seal.

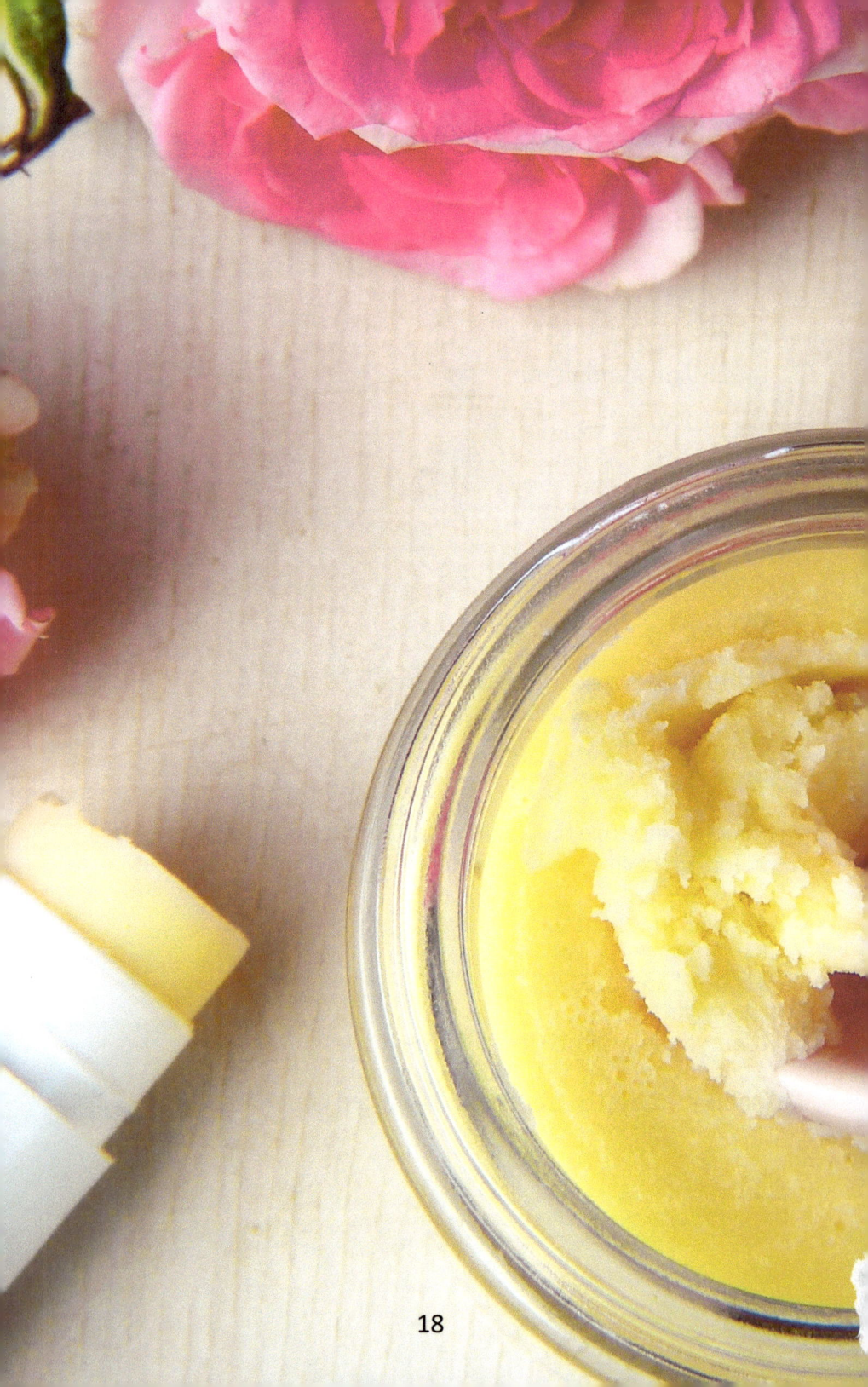

Beeswax Lip Balm

Ingredients

62,5 ml nut oil

1/4 oz beeswax

5 ml honey

5 drops essential oil (never use extracts found in cooking sections as they contain alcohol – use Comfrey, Rosemary, Tea Tree or Camphor Oils)

Few drops beetroot juice

Method

Heat the nut oil and beeswax in a double boiler over boiling water until the beeswax has melted.

Remove the mixture from the heat.

Whip the mixture with an electric beater until creamy.

Add the honey, essential oil and beetroot juice.

Whip the mixture again.

Store the lip gloss / balm in small glass jars.

If the balm is too hard (waxy) add more oil to your mixture.

If the balm is too soft add more wax.

Don't use food colouring as it may contain alcohol base.

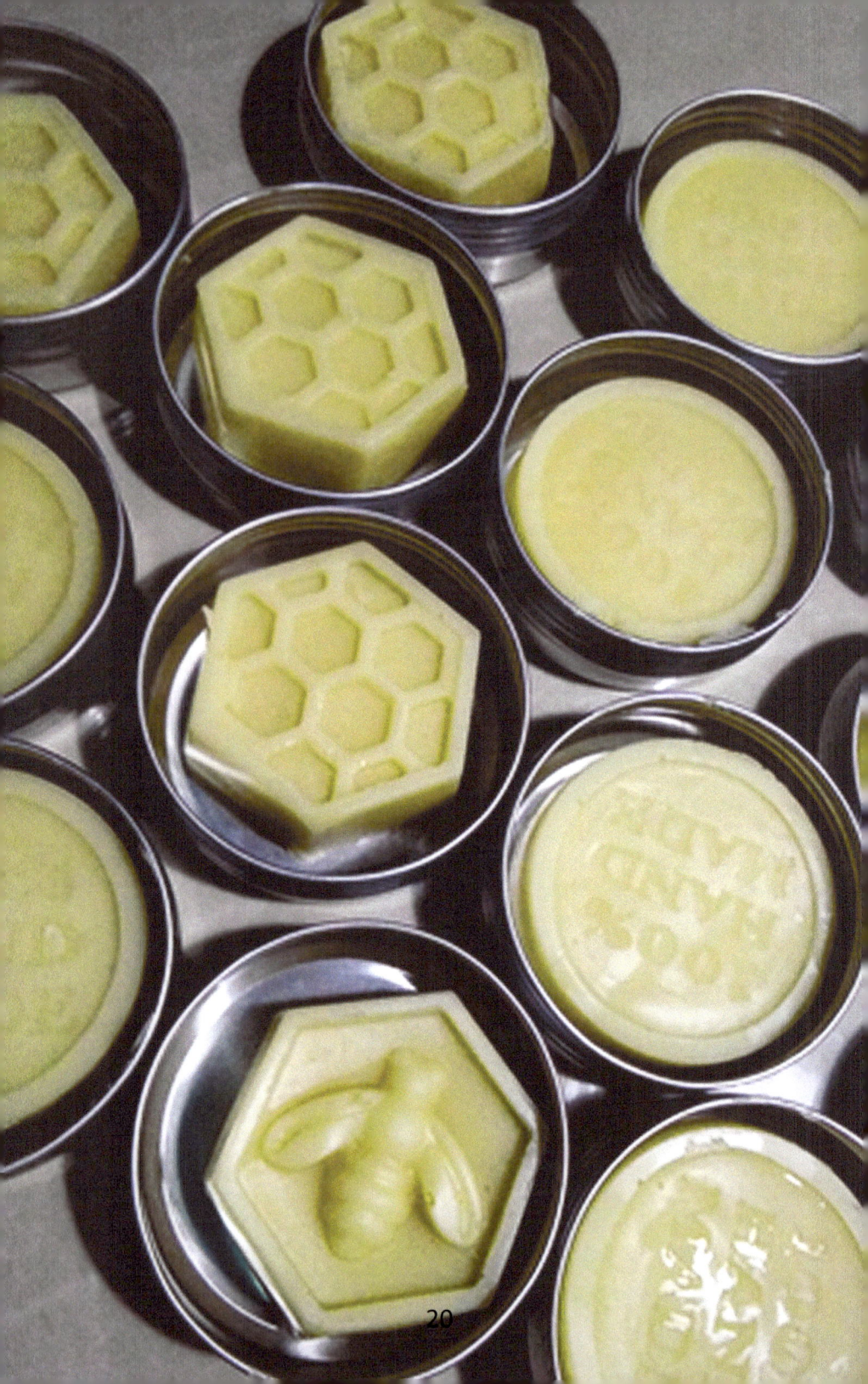

20

Beeswax Lotion Bars

Ingredients

8 oz. beeswax

8 oz. cocoa butter

8 oz. shea butter

Method

Combine the beeswax, cocoa butter and shea butter together in the top of a double boiler over boiling water (see section on melting beeswax).

Mix well.

Remove from the heat.

Pour the melted mixture into molds.

Beeswax Lip Gloss

Ingredients

¾ oz beeswax

6 oz sweet almond oil

10 ml rose essential oil

Method

Melt the beeswax in the top of the double boiler (see section on melting beeswax).

Add the sweet almond oil.

Stir with a spoon.

Remove from the heat.

Leave the mixture to cool slightly.

Add the rose essential oil.

Pour the lip gloss into sterilized containers.

Beeswax Hand Lotion

Ingredients

125 ml beeswax

125 ml coconut oil

75 ml sweet almond oil

166 ml glycerin

Method

Combine the beeswax and coconut oil together in the top of a double boiler over boiling water.

Once the beeswax and coconut oil have melted add the sweet almond oil and glycerin.

Mix well.

Remove from the heat.

Pour the hand lotion into a sterilized container while it is still hot.

Leave the lotion to set.

Honey Body Product Recipes

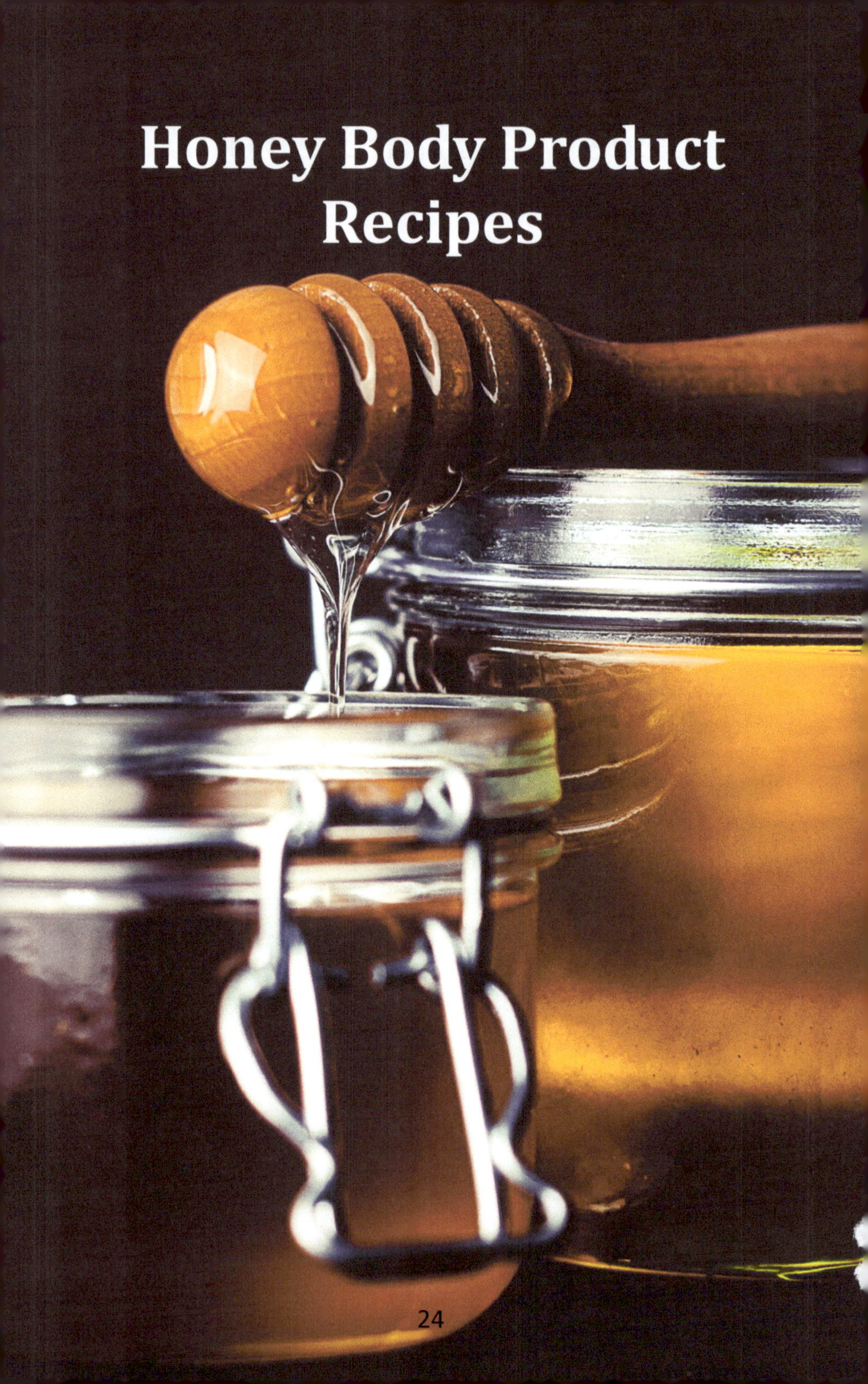

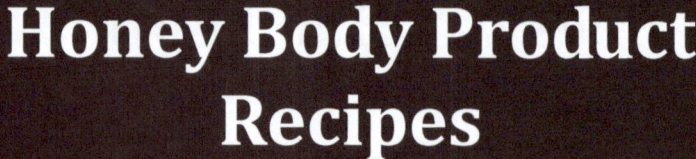

Honey Almond Sugar Scrub

Ingredients

375 ml white sugar

125 ml honey

10 ml almond extract

Method

Combine all the ingredients together.

Mix well.

Pour the mixture into a glass container and seal.

Honey Pistachio Sugar Scrub

Ingredients

500 ml white sugar

125 ml honey

125 ml pistachio oil

Method

Combine all the ingredients together.

Mix well.

Pour the mixture into a glass container and seal.

Honey Apple Face Mask

Ingredients

1 apple (peeled, cored and quartered)

25 ml honey

Method

Blend the apple and honey in a blender until smooth.

Remove the mixture from the blender.

Refrigerate for 10 minutes.

Apply the mixture to your face using a patting motion and be sure to pat until the honey becomes tacky.

Leave it on for 30 minutes.

Rinse with warm water.

Honey Pimple Remedy

Make a paste by mixing 37,5 ml honey and 5 ml cinnamon together.

Apply this paste on the pimples before sleeping.

Wash it off the next morning with warm water.

Repeat for two weeks, pimples will disappear forever.

Avocado Honey Hair Conditioner

Ingredients

1 avocado (peeled, stoned and mashed)

25 ml pure honey

Method

Combine the avocado and honey together.

Blend until smooth.

Smooth the mixture into the hair.

Cover head with wrap or shower cap.

Leave on hair for 20 minutes.

Wash and rinse the hair with warm water.

Honey Hair Conditioner

Ingredients

166 ml hot water

125 ml glycerin

50 ml liquid lecithin

125 ml sage leaves

125 ml pure honey

50 ml buttermilk powder

Method

Combine the water and sage together.

Leave for 15 minutes.

Strain the sage leaves from the liquid.

Combine the sage liquid, glycerin, lecithin, honey and buttermilk powder together.

Mix well.

Massage the mixture into the hair.

Cover head with wrap or shower cap.

Leave for 60 minutes.

Wash and rinse the hair with warm water.

Honey And Banana Hair Mask

Ingredients

1 banana (peeled and mashed)

25 ml pure honey

25 ml plain yogurt

12,5 ml almond oil

Method

Combine the banana, honey, yogurt and almond oil together.

Mix well.

Massage into wet hair.

Cover head with wrap or shower cap.

Leave on hair for 30 minutes.

Wash and rinse the hair.

Honey Hair Mask

Ingredients

50 ml pure honey

25 ml almond oil

25 ml apple cider vinegar

Method

Combine the honey, almond oil and apple cider vinegar together.

Mix well.

Massage into wet hair.

Cover head with wrap or shower cap.

Leave on hair for 30 minutes.

Wash and rinse the hair.

Honey Shampoo

Ingredients

125 ml pure honey

250 ml glycerin

25 ml witch hazel

125 ml rose water

10 ml unscented liquid soap

25 ml alcohol

Method

Combine the honey, glycerin, witch hazel, rose water, liquid soap and alcohol together.

Mix well.

Pour into glass jar.

Use to shampoo your hair as normal.

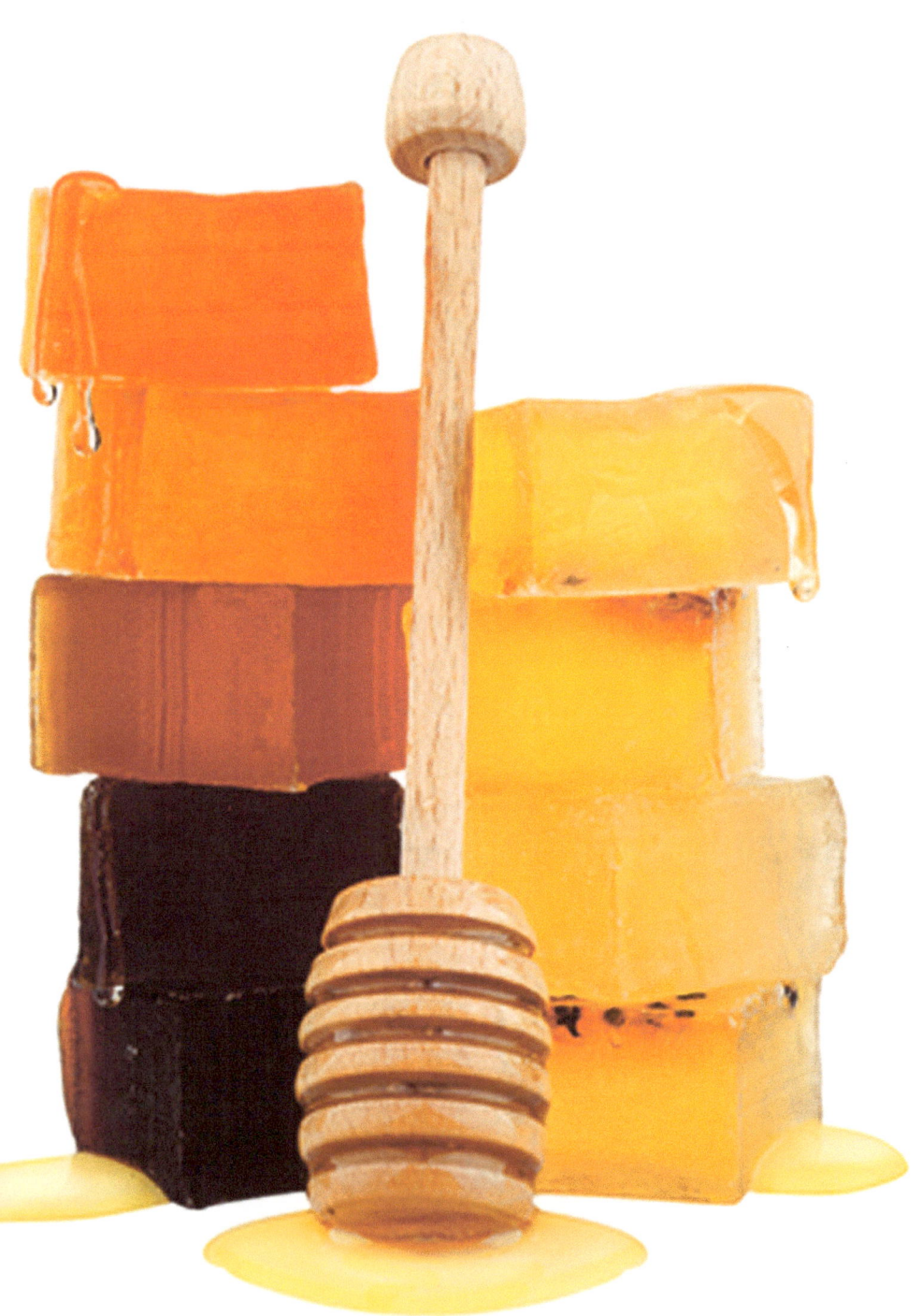

Honey And Glycerin Soap

Ingredients

250 ml unscented glycerin soap

10 ml melted beeswax

10 ml honey

Method

Combine the glycerin soap and beeswax together in the top of a double boiler.

Heat until the soap is liquid.

Stir very well.

Remove the mixture from the heat.

Add the honey.

Mix well.

Pour the honey glycerin soap into molds.

Leave the soap to set.